ONE MEAL A DAY COOKBOOK AFTER 60

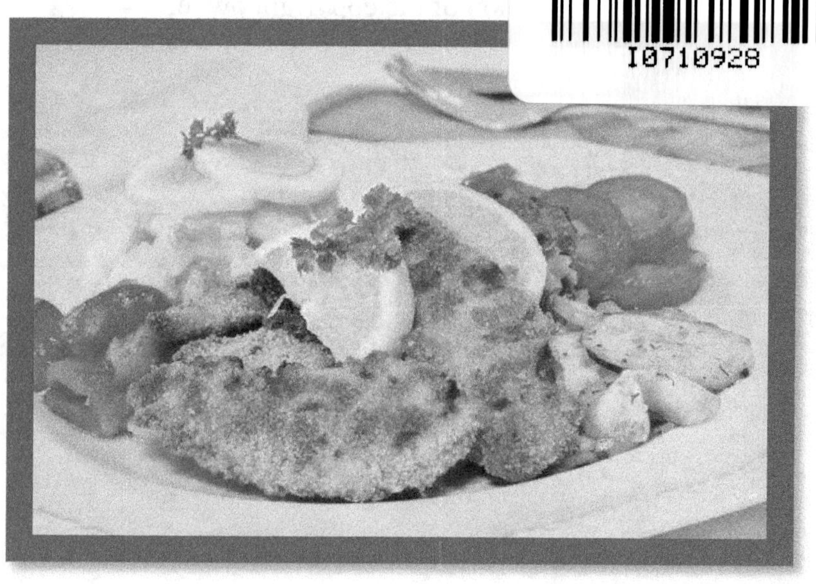

A complete meal plan for staying healthy and active for seniors

EVELYN T. LATTORE

OTHER BOOKS BY PUBLISHER

SMOOTHIE FOR GUT HEALTH

THE SUPER GUT COOKBOOK

FIX YOUR GUT HEALTH

THE BIG DASH COOKBOOK FOR BEGINNERS

20 HEALTHY LOW-CARB RECIPES FOR WEIGHTLOSS

TABLE OF CONTENTS

INTRODUCTION

My grandfather was always a health-conscious person, but in recent years his health began to decline. He started to suffer from chronic pain and fatigue, and he was concerned about his overall health. After consulting with his doctor and doing some research, he decided to try a one meal a day plan to improve his health.

At first, he found it difficult to adjust to the new diet. He was used to eating three meals a day, and he was not sure how he was going to make it through the day with only one meal. But he was determined to give it a try and was willing to make the necessary adjustments in order to improve his health.

My grandfather began to plan his meals carefully. He focused on nutrient-dense foods that would provide him with essential vitamins and minerals. He also made sure to include plenty of lean proteins, complex carbohydrates, and healthy fats. He also included plenty of fruits and vegetables for added fiber and antioxidants.

Once he had his meal plan in place, my grandfather began to stick to it. He ate his one meal each day and made sure to stay hydrated throughout the day by drinking plenty of water. He also began to exercise regularly, which helped to increase his energy levels and keep his body strong.

After consistent lifestyle of eating one meal a day, my grandfather began to notice a difference in his health. He had more energy and was no longer suffering from chronic pain. He also found that he was able to focus better and his mood improved.

My grandfather continued to follow his one meal a day plan and was able to maintain his health improvements. He also found that he was able to save money by sticking to the plan, as he no longer needed to buy as many groceries.

My grandfather's experience with the one meal a day plan was a positive one. He was 70 as at the time and he was able to improve his health, save money, and enjoy the benefits of a healthier lifestyle.

I have made this book a comprehensive cookbook designed to help older adults make healthy and nutritious meals. This cookbook seeks to encourage seniors, and those who care for them, to make home-cooked, delicious meals that are both nutritious and easy to make.

It is designed to provide a wide variety of recipes that are suitable for seniors with different dietary needs and preferences.

I have carefully included recipes for soups, salads, breakfast, lunch, dinner and sea-food. Each recipe is designed to be simple and easy to make, so that seniors don't have to spend hours in the kitchen. I have also carefully prepared a 30 days meal plan to help seniors stay abreast in knowing what to cook.

This book is an excellent resource for seniors who want to make healthy and delicious meals. It also provides a great way for friends and family members to show their support for the elderly by providing healthy and nutritious meals for them. This cookbook is sure to be a hit with seniors and those who care for them.

The Benefits of Eating One Meal A Day After 60

Weight Loss: One meal a day can help you lose weight, as it reduces your calorie consumption and increases the amount of time you spend in a fasted state.

Improved Digestion: Eating one meal a day can help improve digestion and reduce bloating and discomfort. Eating one big meal a day reduces the strain on your digestive system, allowing it to function more efficiently.

Reduced Stress: Eating one meal a day can reduce stress as it simplifies meal planning and preparation, and reduces the number of times you have to think about food throughout the day.

Improved Energy Levels: Eating one meal a day can help improve energy levels, as it reduces the number of times your body has to metabolize food. Eating one large meal may provide a more sustained energy release throughout the day.

Better Mental Clarity: Eating one meal a day can help you focus and stay alert, as it reduces the amount of time you spend digesting food. This can help you think more clearly and remain productive.

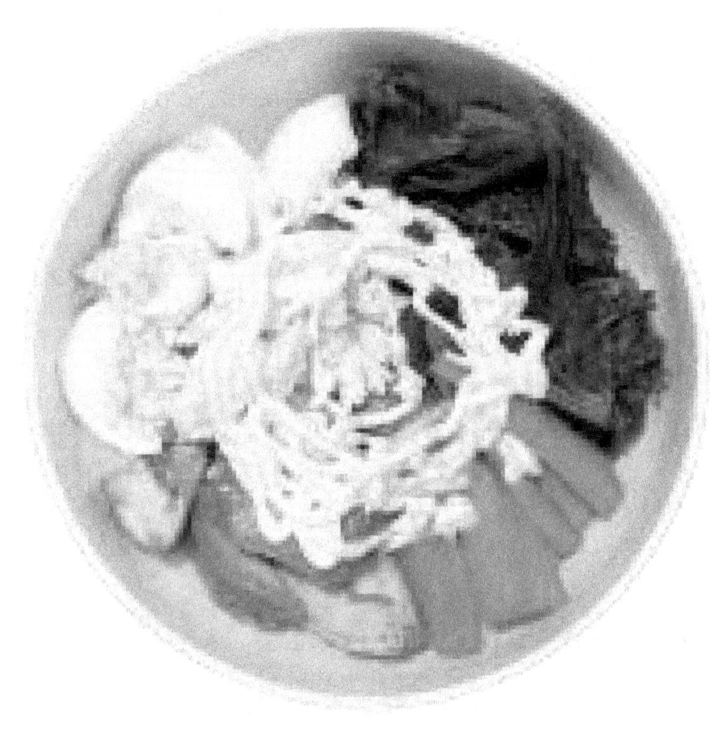

CHAPTER ONE

Essential Vitamins and Minerals for Seniors

As people age, their bodies require different levels of essential vitamins and minerals. Seniors need to be aware of the specific amounts of the nutrients their bodies need in order to stay healthy. Vitamins and minerals are essential for seniors for a variety of reasons.

Not only do they provide essential nutrients for the body, but they also help to maintain strong bones, help to prevent chronic illnesses, and provide a wide range of other health benefits.

Vitamin A is important for seniors because it helps to protect their vision, skin, and immune system. Vitamin A can be found in foods such as carrots, sweet potatoes, spinach, and cantaloupe. Vitamin B is vital for seniors because it helps to maintain energy levels and a healthy central nervous system. Vitamin B can be found in foods such as fish, eggs, and dairy products. Vitamin C is important for seniors as it helps to keep their skin healthy and aids in the absorption of iron. Vitamin C can be found in foods such as oranges, strawberries, and broccoli.

Vitamin D is also important for seniors as it helps to regulate calcium and phosphorus levels in the body. Vitamin D can be found in foods such as dairy products, salmon, and egg yolks.

Minerals are also essential for seniors. Calcium is important for seniors as it helps to maintain strong bones and teeth. Calcium can be found in foods such as dairy products, broccoli, and kale.

Iron is important for seniors as it helps to transport oxygen throughout the body. Iron can be found in foods such as red meat, legumes, and whole grains. Magnesium is important for seniors because it helps to maintain muscle and nerve function. Magnesium can be found in foods such as leafy greens, nuts, and seeds.

Seniors should also be aware of how much of each vitamin and mineral they should be consuming. It is important to note that the recommended daily allowance (RDA) for vitamins and minerals will vary based on age, gender, and other factors. Additionally, seniors should talk to their doctor if they are unsure about the proper levels of vitamins and minerals that they should be consuming.

In conclusion, vitamins and minerals are essential for seniors. They help to protect their vision, skin, and immune system, maintain energy levels, and regulate calcium and phosphorus levels. Seniors should be aware of the specific amounts of the nutrients that their bodies need in order to stay healthy. Additionally, they should talk to their doctor if they are unsure about the proper levels of vitamins and minerals that they should be consuming.

Healthy Eating Habits for Seniors

Healthy eating habits are incredibly important for seniors as they age. Eating nutrient-rich foods, avoiding processed and sugary foods, and staying active can help seniors maintain their health and wellbeing.

With age, seniors need to pay extra attention to their diets to ensure they are getting the vitamins, minerals and other essential nutrients they need to stay healthy.

Seniors should focus on nutrient-dense foods, such as fruits, vegetables, whole grains, lean proteins, and healthy fats. These foods provide vitamins and minerals that can help support seniors' immune systems, boost energy levels, and support healthy bones and muscles. Seniors should limit their intake of processed foods, which are high in unhealthy fats, salt, and added sugars. Eating too many processed foods can lead to weight gain, which can put seniors at risk for heart disease, diabetes, and other serious health issues.

In addition to eating healthy foods, seniors should make sure to stay hydrated by drinking plenty of water. Drinking enough water helps keep the body hydrated, helps flush out toxins, and can help with digestion. Seniors should also pay attention to portion sizes and avoid overeating. Overeating can result in weight gain and other health issues.

Staying physically active is also an important part of maintaining healthy eating habits for seniors. Regular physical activity can help seniors maintain a healthy weight, reduce their risk of chronic diseases, and improve their overall mood and mental health. Physical activity can help seniors stay strong and improve their balance and coordination, reducing their risk of falling.

Most importantly, seniors should look for ways to make healthy eating easier and more enjoyable. This can include planning meals ahead of time, trying new recipes, and making healthy snacks available. Eating with family or friends can also make healthy eating more enjoyable.

Healthy eating habits are essential for seniors as they age. Eating nutrient-rich foods, avoiding processed and sugary foods, staying hydrated and physically active, and making healthy eating enjoyable can help seniors maintain their health and wellbeing. With the right habits, seniors can enjoy a long, healthy life.

Meal Planning Strategies for Seniors

Shop in Bulk: Seniors can save money and reduce trips to the grocery store by purchasing non-perishable items in bulk.

Plan Ahead: Making a meal plan for the week or month can help seniors save money and make sure they are eating a balanced, nutritious diet.

Go for Simple Recipes: Simple recipes with only a few ingredients are a great way for seniors to make healthy meals without spending a lot of time in the kitchen.

Meal Prep: Prepping meals ahead of time can help seniors make sure they have healthy meals when they're busy.

Look for Deals: Taking advantage of special offers and discounts can help seniors stretch their food budget.

Make Use of Leftovers: Making sure to use up leftovers can help seniors save money and reduce food waste.

Join a Food Co-op: Joining a food co-op can help seniors access fresh, locally grown food at a lower cost.

Involve Others: Involving family and friends in meal planning and preparation can help reduce the workload for seniors. Having the extra help can also be beneficial for seniors who may not be able to prepare meals for themselves.

CHAPTER TWO

Breakfast Recipes
Egg Muffins

Ingredients:

6 eggs, ½ cup diced ham, ½ cup diced bell pepper, ¼ cup grated cheese, ½ teaspoon dried oregano.

Method of Preparation:

Preheat oven to 350°F. Grease a 12-cup muffin tin. Beat eggs in a large bowl. Add ham, bell pepper, cheese, and oregano. Mix well. Spoon the mixture into each muffin cup. Bake for 20 minutes.

Time of Preparation: 25 minutes.

Overnight Oats

Ingredients:

1 cup of old-fashioned oats, 1 cup of milk, 2 tablespoons of honey, 1 teaspoon of vanilla extract, 2 tablespoons of chopped almonds or walnuts.

Method of Preparation:

In a bowl, mix oats, milk, honey, and vanilla extract. Place in the refrigerator overnight with a plastic wrap cover. In the morning, stir in the chopped nuts. Serve cold or heat in the microwave for a warm breakfast.

Time of Preparation: 10 minutes.

Apple Cinnamon Pancakes

Ingredients:

2 cups whole-wheat flour, 2 teaspoons baking powder, ¼ teaspoon ground cinnamon, 1 teaspoon salt, 1 cup milk, 2 tablespoons olive oil, 2 tablespoons honey, 1 egg, 1 cup diced apples.

Method of Preparation:

In a bowl, mix together the flour, baking powder, cinnamon, and salt. In a separate bowl, mix together the milk, olive oil, honey, and egg. After adding the liquid components, stir the dry ingredients just until combined.

The apple cubes are folded in. Spray nonstick cooking spray in a skillet that is already heated to medium heat. Using a ¼ cup measuring cup, scoop the pancake batter onto the skillet. Flip after cooking for 2 to 3 minutes till golden brown. Cook for an additional 2-3 minutes. Serve warm with maple syrup. ***Time of Preparation: 20 minutes.***

Yogurt Parfait

Ingredients:

2 cups plain Greek yogurt, 1 cup mixed berries, ¼ cup granola, 2 tablespoons honey.

Method of Preparation:

In a bowl, mix together the yogurt, honey, and berries. Layer the yogurt mixture, granola, and berries into a parfait glass. Top with additional berries and honey, if desired. Serve cold. ***Time of Preparation: 5 minutes.***

Banana-Berry Smoothie

Ingredients:

1 frozen banana, ½ cup frozen berries, 1 cup almond milk, 1 tablespoon honey.

Method of Preparation:

In a blender, combine banana, berries, almond milk, and honey. Blend until smooth. Serve cold.

Time of Preparation: 5 minutes.

Avocado Toast

Ingredients:

2 slices whole-wheat bread, 1 avocado, 1 tablespoon olive oil, 2 tablespoons feta cheese, salt and pepper to taste.

Method of Preparation:

Toast the bread slices. Slice the avocado and place on the toasted bread slices. Add feta cheese and drizzle with olive oil. Add salt and pepper to taste.

Time of Preparation: 5 minutes.

Peanut Butter and Banana Sandwich

Ingredients:

2 slices whole-wheat bread, 2 tablespoons peanut butter, 1 banana, sliced.

Method of Preparation:

Spread peanut butter on one slice of bread. Put the slices of banana on top of the peanut butter. Top with the other slice of bread. Cut in half and serve.

Time of Preparation: 5 minutes.

Oatmeal with Fresh Fruit

Ingredients:

1 cup rolled oats, 1 cup water, 1 cup fresh fruit (blueberries, strawberries, apples, etc.), 2 tablespoons honey or maple syrup.

Method of Preparation:

In a saucepan, bring the water to a boil. Turn the heat down to low after adding the oats. Cook for 5 minutes, stirring occasionally.

Put the honey or maple syrup in after taking the pan off the heat. Divide the oatmeal into two bowls and top with the fresh fruit. Serve warm.

Time of Preparation: 10 minutes.

Veggie Scramble

Ingredients:

2 eggs, 1 cup diced vegetables (onion, bell peppers, mushrooms, etc.), ¼ cup grated cheese, salt and pepper to taste.

Method of Preparation:

Spray nonstick cooking spray into a skillet that is already hot over medium heat. Add the vegetables and sauté for 3-4 minutes until softened. Crack the eggs into the skillet.

Stir constantly and cook for 3-4 minutes until the eggs are cooked through. add the shredded cheese, a pinch of salt, and pepper. Serve warm.

Time of Preparation: 10 minutes.

English Muffin with Fried Egg

Ingredients:

1 whole-wheat English muffin, 1 egg, 1 teaspoon olive oil, 1 tablespoon grated cheese, salt and pepper to taste.

Method of Preparation:

Heat a skillet over medium heat and add the olive oil. Crack the egg into the skillet and cook for 3-4 minutes until the egg is cooked through. Toast the English muffin. Place the egg on top of the muffin and sprinkle with grated cheese, salt and pepper to taste. Serve warm.

Time of Preparation: 5 minutes.

Protein Fruit Bowl

Ingredients:

1 scoop vanilla protein powder, 1 cup yogurt, 1 cup fresh fruit (blueberries, strawberries, bananas, etc.), 1 tablespoon chopped nuts.

Method of Preparation:

In a bowl, combine the protein powder, yogurt, and fruit. Top with chopped nuts. Serve cold or at room temperature. *Time of Preparation: 5 minutes.*

French Toast

Ingredients:

2 slices whole-wheat bread, 2 eggs, 1 tablespoon milk, ½ teaspoon ground cinnamon, 2 tablespoons maple syrup, 1 teaspoon butter.

Method of Preparation:

In a shallow bowl, whisk together the eggs, milk, and cinnamon. Dip each slice of bread into the egg mixture, ensuring both sides are evenly coated. Butter is added to a skillet that is already hot.

The bread slices should be cooked in the skillet for two to three minutes on each side to get golden brown. Serve with maple syrup.

Time of Preparation: 10 minutes.

Egg and Turkey Bacon Sandwich

Ingredients:

2 slices whole-wheat bread, 2 eggs, 2 slices turkey bacon, 1 tablespoon butter, 2 slices cheese, salt and pepper to taste.

Method of Preparation:

Heat a skillet over medium heat and add the butter. Crack the eggs into the skillet and cook for 3-4 minutes until the eggs are cooked through. Cook the turkey bacon in a different skillet in the interim.

Toast the bread slices. Assemble the sandwich with the eggs, bacon, and cheese. Add salt and pepper to taste. Serve warm.

Time of Preparation: 10 minutes.

Breakfast Burrito

Ingredients:

2 eggs, 1 cup diced vegetables (onion, bell peppers, mushrooms, etc.), 2 tablespoons grated cheese, 1 whole-wheat tortilla, salt and pepper to taste.

Method of Preparation:

Heat a skillet over medium heat and spray with non-stick cooking spray. Add the vegetables and sauté for 3-4 minutes until softened. Crack the eggs into the skillet.

Stir constantly and cook for 3-4 minutes until the eggs are cooked through. add the shredded cheese, a pinch of salt, and pepper. Place the egg mixture onto the tortilla and roll into a burrito. Serve warm.

Time of Preparation: 10 minutes.

Breakfast Quesadilla

Ingredients:

2 whole-wheat tortillas, 1 cup grated cheese, 2 eggs, 2 tablespoons salsa, 2 tablespoons chopped cilantro.

Method of Preparation:

Heat a skillet over medium heat and spray with non-stick cooking spray. Crack the eggs into the skillet and cook for 3-4 minutes until the eggs are cooked through. Place one tortilla onto the skillet and top with half of the grated cheese. Spread the egg mixture and salsa onto the cheese.

Add the second tortilla and the remaining cheese on top. Cook for 3-4 minutes until the cheese is melted and the tortilla is golden brown. Cut into wedges and top with chopped cilantro. Serve warm.

Time of Preparation: 10 minutes.

Baked Oatmeal

Ingredients:

2 cups old-fashioned oats, 2 cups almond milk, 1 teaspoon ground cinnamon, 2 tablespoons honey, 1 teaspoon vanilla extract, ½ cup diced apples, ½ cup chopped walnuts, 2 tablespoons melted butter.

Method of Preparation:

Preheat oven to 350°F. In a bowl, mix together the oats, almond milk, cinnamon, honey, and vanilla extract. Stir in the apples and walnuts. In a greased 9 x 13-inch baking dish, pour the ingredients. Drizzle with melted butter. Bake for 30 minutes. Serve warm.

Time of Preparation: 35 minutes.

Egg and Cheese Muffins

Ingredients:

6 eggs, ½ cup diced ham, ½ cup diced bell pepper, ¼ cup grated cheese, ½ teaspoon dried oregano.

Method of Preparation:

Preheat oven to 350°F. Grease a 12-cup muffin tin. Beat eggs in a large bowl. Add ham, bell pepper, cheese, and oregano. Mix well. Spoon the mixture into each muffin cup. Bake for 20 minutes.

Time of Preparation: 25 minutes.

Fruit and Yogurt Parfait

Ingredients:

2 cups plain Greek yogurt, 1 cup mixed berries, ¼ cup granola, 2 tablespoons honey.

Method of Preparation:

In a bowl, mix together the yogurt, honey, and berries. Layer the yogurt mixture, granola, and berries into a parfait glass. Top with additional berries and honey, if desired. Serve cold. *Time of Preparation: 5 minutes.*

Egg and Spinach Sandwich

Ingredients:

2 slices whole-wheat bread, 2 eggs, 2 cups fresh spinach, 2 slices cheese, 1 tablespoon butter, salt and pepper to taste.

Method of Preparation:

Heat a skillet over medium heat and add the butter. Crack the eggs into the skillet and cook for 3-4 minutes until the eggs are cooked through. Meanwhile, sauté the spinach in a separate skillet for 3-4 minutes until wilted.

Toast the bread slices. Assemble the sandwich with the eggs, spinach, and cheese. Add salt and pepper to taste. Serve warm.

Time of Preparation: 10 minutes.

CHAPTER THREE

Lunch Recipes

Vegetable Soup:

Ingredients:

4 cups of vegetable broth, 2 cups of diced potatoes, 1 cup of diced carrots, 1/2 cup of diced celery, 1/4 cup of chopped onion, 1/4 teaspoon of garlic powder, 1/4 teaspoon of pepper, 1/4 teaspoon of dried parsley, 1/4 teaspoon of dried oregano.

Method of Preparation:

In a large pot, combine vegetable broth, potatoes, carrots, celery, and onion. Cook for 15 minutes, stirring regularly, after bringing to a boil, stirring occasionally.

Add garlic powder, pepper, parsley, and oregano. Simmer for another 20 minutes until vegetables are tender. Serve hot.

Time of Preparation: 35 minutes.

Quinoa Bowl:

Ingredients:

1 cup of cooked quinoa, 1/2 cup of diced bell peppers, 1/2 cup of diced zucchini, 1/4 cup of diced red onion, 1/4 cup of canned black beans, 1/4 cup of corn kernels, 2 tablespoons of olive oil, 1 tablespoon of red wine vinegar, 1/4 teaspoon of salt, and 1/4 teaspoon of pepper.

Method of Preparation:

In a large bowl, combine cooked quinoa, bell peppers, zucchini, red onion, black beans, and corn kernels. Mix the olive oil, red wine vinegar, salt, and pepper in a small bowl. Toss the quinoa mixture with the dressing after pouring it over it. Serve immediately.

Egg Salad Sandwich:

Ingredients:

3 hard-boiled eggs, 1/4 cup of mayonnaise, 1/4 cup of diced celery, 1 tablespoon of chopped parsley, 1/4 teaspoon of salt, and 1/4 teaspoon of pepper.

Method of Preparation:

In a medium bowl, mash hard-boiled eggs with a fork. Add mayonnaise, celery, parsley, salt, and pepper. Mix until everything is well combined. Serve on your favorite bread.

Time of Preparation: 10 minutes.

Baked Salmon:

Ingredients:

2 salmon fillets, 2 tablespoons of butter, 1 tablespoon of lemon juice, 1/4 teaspoon of garlic powder, 1/4 teaspoon of paprika, 1/4 teaspoon of salt, and 1/4 teaspoon of pepper.

Method of Preparation:

Preheat oven to 375°F. Place salmon fillets in a baking dish and top with butter and lemon juice. Add paprika, salt, pepper, and garlic powder. Bake the fish for 15 to 20 minutes, or until done. Serve with your favorite vegetables.

Time of Preparation: 20 minutes.

Baked Chicken:

Ingredients:

2 boneless, skinless chicken breasts, 2 tablespoons of olive oil, 1 tablespoon of Italian seasoning, 1/4 teaspoon of garlic powder, 1/4 teaspoon of salt, and 1/4 teaspoon of pepper.

Method of Preparation:

Preheat oven to 375°F. Place chicken breasts in a baking dish and top with olive oil. Salt, pepper, garlic powder, and Italian seasoning should be added. Bake for 20-25 minutes until chicken is cooked through. Serve with your favorite vegetables.

Time of Preparation: 25 minutes.

Tuna Salad:

Ingredients:

2 cans of tuna, 1/4 cup of diced celery, 1/4 cup of diced onion, 1/4 cup of mayonnaise, 1 tablespoon of lemon juice, 1/4 teaspoon of salt, and 1/4 teaspoon of pepper.

Method of Preparation:

In a medium bowl, combine tuna, celery, onion, mayonnaise, lemon juice, salt, and pepper. Mix until everything is well combined. Serve on your favorite bread.

Time of Preparation: 10 minutes.

Roasted Vegetables:

Ingredients:

1 cup of diced potatoes, 1 cup of diced carrots, 1 cup of diced bell peppers, 2 tablespoons of olive oil, 1/4 teaspoon of garlic powder, 1/4 teaspoon of salt, and 1/4 teaspoon of pepper.

Method of Preparation:

Preheat oven to 375°F. Place potatoes, carrots, and bell peppers in a baking dish and top with olive oil. Sprinkle with garlic powder, salt, and pepper. Vegetables should be soft after 25 to 30 minutes in the oven. Serve warm.

Time of Preparation: 30 minutes.

Greek Yogurt Parfait:

Ingredients:

1 cup of plain Greek yogurt, 1/2 cup of granola, 1/2 cup of diced strawberries, 1/2 cup of diced blueberries, 1/4 cup of chopped almonds.

Method of Preparation:

In a bowl or glass, layer Greek yogurt, granola, strawberries, blueberries, and almonds. Serve cold.

Time of Preparation: 10 minutes.

Grilled Cheese Sandwich:

Ingredients:

2 slices of bread, 2 tablespoons of butter, 2 slices of cheddar cheese.

Method of Preparation:

Heat a skillet over medium heat. Each slice of bread should have butter spread on one side. Place one slice of bread butter side down in the skillet. Top with cheddar cheese and the other slice of bread butter side up. Cook for 3-4 minutes until bread is golden brown and cheese is melted. Serve warm.

Time of Preparation: 10 minutes.

BLT Sandwich:

Ingredients:

2 slices of bread, 2 pieces of bacon, 1 tomato, 1 lettuce leaf, and 2 tablespoons of mayonnaise

Method of Preparation:

Heat a skillet over medium heat and cook bacon for 3-4 minutes until crispy. Spread mayonnaise on one side of each slice of bread. One slice of bread should be placed in the skillet mayonnaise side down.

Add a lettuce leaf, tomato, and bacon on top. Add the second slice of bread on top, mayonnaise side up. Fry the bread for 3 to 4 minutes, or until golden brown. Serve warm.

Time of Preparation: 10 minutes.

Egg Fried Rice:

Ingredients:

1 cup of cooked white rice, 2 tablespoons of butter, 2 eggs, 1/4 cup of diced onion, 1/4 cup of diced bell peppers, 1/4 cup of diced carrots, 1/4 teaspoon of garlic powder, 1/4 teaspoon of salt, and 1/4 teaspoon of pepper.

Method of Preparation:

Heat a large skillet over medium heat. Add butter and eggs and cook for 2-3 minutes until eggs are scrambled. Add onion, bell peppers, carrots, garlic powder, salt, and pepper. Cook for an additional 3-4 minutes until vegetables are tender. Add cooked rice and stir to combine. Sauté for a further 2 to 3 minutes, or until everything is well heated. Serve warm.

Time of Preparation: 10 minutes.

Baked Sweet Potato:

Ingredients:

1 large sweet potato, 2 tablespoons of olive oil, 1/4 teaspoon of salt, and 1/4 teaspoon of pepper.

Method of Preparation:

Preheat oven to 375°F. Pierce sweet potato with a fork several times and place on a baking sheet. Top with olive oil, salt, and pepper. Bake for 45-50 minutes until potato is fork tender. Serve warm.

Time of Preparation: 50 minutes.

Chicken Salad:

Ingredients:

2 cups of diced cooked chicken, 1/4 cup of diced celery, 1/4 cup of diced onion, 1/4 cup of mayonnaise, 1 tablespoon of lemon juice, 1/4 teaspoon of salt, and 1/4 teaspoon of pepper.

Method of Preparation:

In a bowl, combine chicken, celery, onion, mayonnaise, lemon juice, salt, and pepper. Mix until everything is well combined. Serve on your favorite bread.

Time of Preparation: 10 minutes.

Green Smoothie:

Ingredients:

1 cup of spinach, 1 banana, 1/2 cup of diced pineapple, 1/2 cup of almond milk, 1 tablespoon of honey.

Method of Preparation:

Place spinach, banana, pineapple, almond milk, and honey in a blender and blend until smooth. Serve cold.

Time of Preparation: 5 minutes.

Roasted Chicken:

Ingredients:

2 boneless, skinless chicken breasts, 2 tablespoons of olive oil, 1 tablespoon of Italian seasoning, 1/4 teaspoon of garlic powder, 1/4 teaspoon of salt, and 1/4 teaspoon of pepper.

Method of Preparation:

Preheat oven to 375°F. Place chicken breasts in a baking dish and top with olive oil. Add salt, pepper, garlic powder, and Italian seasoning. Chicken should be cooked through in the oven for 20 to 25 minutes. Serve with your favorite vegetables.

Time of Preparation: 25 minutes.

Baked Fish:

Ingredients:

2 fillets of your favorite fish, 2 tablespoons of butter, 2 tablespoons of lemon juice, 1/4 teaspoon of garlic powder, 1/4 teaspoon of salt, and 1/4 teaspoon of pepper.

Method of Preparation:

Preheat oven to 375°F. Place fish fillets in a baking dish and top with butter and lemon juice. Sprinkle with garlic powder, salt, and pepper. Bake the fish for 15 to 20 minutes, or until done. Serve with your favorite vegetables.

Time of Preparation: 20 minutes.

Lentil Soup:

Ingredients:

4 cups of vegetable broth, 1 cup of cooked lentils, 1/2 cup of diced celery, 1/2 cup of diced carrots, 1/4 cup of diced onion, 1/4 teaspoon of garlic powder, 1/4 teaspoon of salt, 1/4 teaspoon of pepper, and 1/4 teaspoon of dried parsley.

Method of Preparation:

In a large pot, combine vegetable broth, lentils, celery, carrots, and onion. Cook for 15 minutes, stirring regularly, after bringing to a boil. Add garlic powder, salt, pepper, and parsley. Simmer for another 20 minutes until vegetables are tender. Serve hot.

Time of Preparation: 35 minutes.

Hummus Sandwich:
Ingredients:

2 slices of bread, 1/4 cup of hummus, 1/2 cup of diced cucumber, 1/4 cup of diced red onion, 2 slices of tomato.

Method of Preparation:

Spread hummus on one side of each slice of bread. Top one slice of bread with cucumber, red onion, and tomato. Place the other slice of bread on top. Serve immediately.

Time of Preparation: 10 minutes.

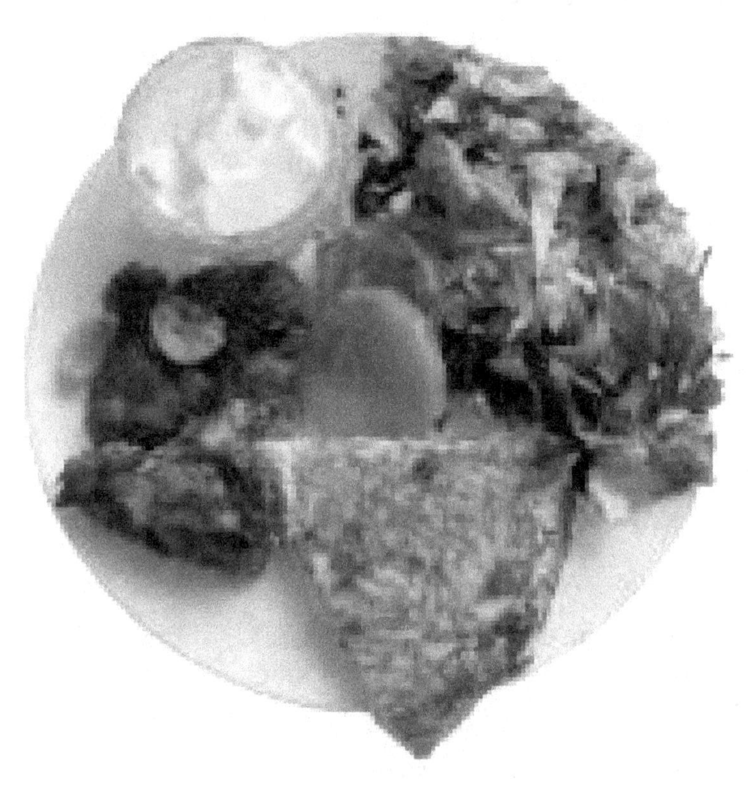

CHAPTER FOUR

Dinner recipes

Baked Salmon with Asparagus and Rice:

Ingredients:

2 salmon fillets, 1 bunch of asparagus, 2 cups of cooked brown rice, 2 tablespoons of olive oil, 1 tablespoon of garlic powder, 1 tablespoon of lemon juice, salt and pepper to taste.

Method:

Preheat oven to 375°F. On a baking sheet covered with parchment paper, arrange the salmon fillets. Add a drizzle of olive oil and season with salt, pepper, garlic powder, and lemon juice.

Place the asparagus around the salmon. Bake for 20 minutes. Serve with cooked brown rice.

Time: 20 minutes.

Spinach Quiche with Sweet Potato Crust:

Ingredients:

2 cups of cooked sweet potato, 1 tablespoon of olive oil, 2 cups of fresh spinach, 1/2 cup of grated cheese, 2 eggs, 1/4 cup of milk, Salt and pepper to taste, along with 1/2 teaspoon each of garlic powder and paprika.

Method:

Preheat oven to 375°F. Spread some olive oil in a 9-inch pie plate. Mash the cooked sweet potato in a bowl, then press into the prepared pie dish. Bake for 15 minutes. In a separate bowl, whisk together eggs, milk, garlic powder, paprika, salt and pepper. On the sweet potato crust, pour the egg mixture. Top with spinach and grated cheese. Bake for 20 minutes.

Time: 35 minutes.

Baked Cod with Garlic and Herb Sauce:

Ingredients:

2 cod fillets, 2 tablespoons of olive oil, 1 tablespoon of garlic powder, 1 teaspoon of dried oregano, 1 teaspoon of dried basil, 2 tablespoons of butter, Salt and pepper, 1/4 cup white wine.

Method:

Preheat oven to 375°F. Place cod fillets on a parchment paper-lined baking sheet. Add a drizzle of olive oil and season with salt, pepper, garlic powder, oregano, and basil. For 15 minutes, bake. Melt the butter in a small pan over medium heat. After the white wine has decreased by half, add it. Pour sauce over the cod and bake for an additional 5 minutes.

Time: 20 minutes.

Baked Chicken Breasts with Mushrooms and Artichokes:

Ingredients:

4 chicken breasts, 6 ounces of sliced mushrooms, 1 can of artichoke hearts, 2 tablespoons of olive oil, 1 tablespoon of garlic powder, 1/2 teaspoon of dried thyme, 2 tablespoons of butter, 1/4 cup of white wine, salt and pepper to taste.

Method:

Preheat oven to 375°F. On a baking sheet covered with parchment paper, arrange the chicken breasts. Drizzle with olive oil and season with garlic powder, thyme, salt and pepper. Top with mushrooms and artichoke hearts. Bake for 20 minutes.

In a small pan over medium heat, melt the butter. Cook white wine after adding it till it has been cut in half. Pour sauce over the chicken and bake for an additional 5 minutes.

Time: 25 minutes.

Veggie Lasagna:

Ingredients:

2 cups of cooked lasagna noodles, 2 cups of ricotta cheese, 2 cups of grated mozzarella cheese, 1 can of diced tomatoes, 1 cup of frozen spinach, 1/2 cup of sliced mushrooms, 1/2 cup of chopped bell pepper, 1/4 cup of grated parmesan cheese, 2 tablespoons of olive oil, 1 tablespoon of garlic powder, 1 teaspoon of dried oregano, salt and pepper to taste.

Method:

Preheat oven to 375°F. Use olive oil to grease a 9-inch baking dish. Layer the cooked lasagna noodles on the bottom of the dish. Top with ricotta cheese, mozzarella cheese, diced tomatoes, spinach, mushrooms, bell pepper, parmesan cheese, garlic powder, oregano, salt and pepper. Bake for 25 minutes.

Time: 30 minutes.

Stuffed Peppers:

Ingredients:

4 bell peppers, 1/2 cup of cooked quinoa, 1/2 cup of cooked black beans, 1/2 cup of corn kernels, 1/4 cup of grated cheese, 2 tablespoons of olive oil, 1 tablespoon of garlic powder, 1 teaspoon of ground cumin, 1/4 cup of salsa, salt and pepper to taste.

Method:

Preheat oven to 375°F. Cut the bell peppers in half, lengthwise. Place on a parchment paper-lined baking sheet. In a bowl, mix together quinoa, black beans, corn kernels, grated cheese, olive oil, garlic powder, cumin, salsa, salt and pepper. Stuff the pepper halves with the mixture. Bake for 20 minutes.

Time: 25 minutes.

Baked Salmon with Lemon Butter Sauce:

Ingredients:

2 salmon fillets, 2 tablespoons of butter, 1 tablespoon of garlic powder, 1/4 cup of white wine, 2 tablespoons of lemon juice, salt and pepper to taste.

Method:

Preheat oven to 375°F. Put the salmon fillets on a baking pan covered with parchment paper. Drizzle with butter and season with garlic powder, salt and pepper. Bake for 15 minutes.

In a small saucepan, heat white wine and lemon juice over medium heat. Cook until reduced by half. Pour sauce over the salmon and bake for an additional 5 minutes.

Time: 20 minutes.

Baked Zucchini with Tomatoes and Feta Cheese:

Ingredients:

2 zucchini, 2 tomatoes, 1/4 cup of feta cheese, 2 tablespoons of olive oil, 1 tablespoon of garlic powder, 1/2 teaspoon of dried oregano, salt and pepper to taste.

Method:

Preheat oven to 375°F. Slice the zucchini and tomatoes and place on a parchment paper-lined baking sheet. Sprinkle with salt, pepper, oregano, garlic powder, and olive oil. Top with feta cheese. Bake for 15 minutes.

Time: 15 minutes.

Baked Salmon with Mango Salsa:
Ingredients:

2 salmon fillets, 1/2 cup of diced mango, 1/4 cup of diced red onion, 1/4 cup of diced red bell pepper, 2 tablespoons of olive oil, 1 tablespoon of garlic powder, 2 tablespoons of lime juice, salt and pepper to taste.

Method:

Preheat oven to 375°F. Salmon fillets should be put on a baking pan covered with parchment paper. Add a drizzle of olive oil and season with salt, pepper, and garlic powder. Add a drizzle of olive oil and season with salt, pepper, and garlic powder. Bake for 15 minutes. In a bowl, mix together mango, red onion, red bell pepper, lime juice, salt and pepper. Serve the mango salsa alongside the fish.

Time: 20 minutes.

Baked Halibut with Roasted Asparagus:

Ingredients:

2 halibut fillets, 1 bunch of asparagus, 2 tablespoons of olive oil, 1 tablespoon of garlic powder, 2 tablespoons of lemon juice, salt and pepper to taste.

Method:

Preheat oven to 375°F. Place halibut fillets on a parchment paper-lined baking sheet. Add a drizzle of olive oil and season with salt, pepper, garlic powder, and lemon juice. Place the asparagus around the halibut. Bake for 20 minutes.

Time: 20 minutes.

Baked Eggplant Parmesan:

Ingredients:

1 large eggplant, 1/2 cup of grated cheese, 1/2 cup of marinara sauce, 2 tablespoons of olive oil, 1 tablespoon of garlic powder, 1/2 teaspoon of dried oregano, salt and pepper to taste.

Method:

Preheat oven to 375°F. Slice the eggplant into 1/4-inch thick slices and place on a parchment paper-lined baking sheet. Add a drizzle of olive oil and season with salt, pepper, garlic powder, and lemon juice. Top with grated cheese and marinara sauce. Bake for 25 minutes.

Time: 25 minutes.

Baked Tofu with Cashews and Broccoli:

Ingredients:

1 block of tofu, 2 cups of broccoli florets, 1/2 cup of roasted cashews, 2 tablespoons of olive oil, 1 tablespoon of garlic powder, 1 teaspoon of ground ginger, salt and pepper to taste.

Method:

Preheat oven to 375°F. Slice the tofu into 1/2-inch thick slices and place on a parchment paper-lined baking sheet. Drizzle with olive oil and season with garlic powder, ground ginger, salt and pepper. Top with cashews and broccoli. Bake for 25 minutes.

Time: 25 minutes.

Baked Cod with Tomatoes and Olives:

Ingredients:

2 cod fillets, 2 tomatoes, 1/4 cup of sliced olives, 2 tablespoons of olive oil, 1 tablespoon of garlic powder, 1/2 teaspoon of dried oregano, salt and pepper to taste.

Method:

Preheat oven to 375°F. Place cod fillets on a parchment paper-lined baking sheet. Sprinkle with salt, pepper, oregano, garlic powder, and olive oil. Top with tomatoes and olives. Bake for 15 minutes.

Time: 15 minutes.

Baked Chicken Fajitas:

Ingredients:

4 chicken breasts, 1 bell pepper, 1 onion, 2 tablespoons of olive oil, 1 tablespoon of garlic powder, 1 teaspoon of ground cumin, 1/2 teaspoon of chili powder, 1/4 cup of salsa, salt and pepper to taste.

Method:

Preheat oven to 375°F. Slice the chicken breasts into 1/2-inch thick strips and place on a parchment paper-lined baking sheet. Drizzle with olive oil and season with garlic powder, cumin, chili powder, salt and pepper. Place the bell pepper and onion on the sheet and bake for 20 minutes. Serve with salsa.

Time: 20 minutes.

Baked Pork Chops with Apples:

Ingredients:

4 pork chops, 2 apples, 2 tablespoons of olive oil, 1 tablespoon of garlic powder, 1/2 teaspoon of dried thyme, 2 tablespoons of butter, 1/4 cup of white wine, salt and pepper to taste.

Method:

Preheat oven to 375°F. On a baking sheet covered with parchment-lined paper, arrange the pork chops. Drizzle with olive oil and season with garlic powder, thyme, salt and pepper. Top with apples. Bake for 15 minutes.

Melt butter in a small pan over medium heat. After the white wine has decreased by half, add it. Pour sauce over the pork chops and bake for an additional 5 minutes.

Time: 20 minutes.

Baked Halibut with Spinach and Feta:

Ingredients:

2 halibut fillets, 2 cups of fresh spinach, 1/4 cup of feta cheese, 2 tablespoons of olive oil, 1 tablespoon of garlic powder, 1/2 teaspoon of dried oregano, salt and pepper to taste.

Method:

Preheat oven to 375°F. Place halibut fillets on a parchment paper-lined baking sheet. Sprinkle with salt, pepper, oregano, garlic powder, and olive oil. Top with spinach and feta cheese. Bake for 15 minutes.

Time: 15 minutes.

Baked Mac and Cheese:

Ingredients:

8 ounces of cooked macaroni noodles, 1 cup of grated cheese, 1/2 cup of milk, 2 tablespoons of butter, 1 tablespoon of garlic powder, 1/2 teaspoon of dried thyme, 1/4 cup of breadcrumbs, salt and pepper to taste.

Method:

Preheat oven to 375°F. Grease a 9-inch baking dish with butter. Place the cooked macaroni noodles in the dish. Top with grated cheese, milk, butter, garlic powder, thyme, salt and pepper. Sprinkle with breadcrumbs. Bake for 25 minutes.

Time: 25 minutes.

Baked Cod with Lemon and Parsley:

Ingredients:

2 cod fillets, 2 tablespoons of butter, 1 tablespoon of garlic powder, 2 tablespoons of lemon juice, 1 tablespoon of chopped fresh parsley, salt and pepper to taste.

Method:

Preheat oven to 375°F. Place cod fillets on a parchment paper-lined baking sheet. Drizzle with butter and season with garlic powder, lemon juice, parsley, salt and pepper. Bake for 15 minutes.

Time: 15 minutes.

Baked Chicken with Sweet Potatoes:

Ingredients:

4 chicken breasts, 2 sweet potatoes, 2 tablespoons of olive oil, 1 tablespoon of garlic powder, 1/2 teaspoon of ground cumin, 1/4 teaspoon of chili powder, salt and pepper to taste.

Method:

Preheat oven to 375°F. On a baking sheet covered with parchment paper, arrange the chicken breasts. Drizzle with olive oil and season with garlic powder, cumin, chili powder, salt and pepper. Place the sweet potatoes around the chicken. Bake for 20 minutes.

Time: 20 minutes.

Baked Fish Tacos:

Ingredients:

2 fish fillets, 8 corn tortillas, 1/4 cup of diced tomatoes, 1/4 cup of diced red onion, 1/4 cup of diced bell pepper, 2 tablespoons of olive oil, 1 tablespoon of garlic powder, 1/4 cup of salsa, salt and pepper to taste.

Method:

Preheat oven to 375°F. Place fish fillets on a parchment paper-lined baking sheet. Add a drizzle of olive oil and season with salt, pepper, and garlic powder.

Bake for 15 minutes. In a bowl, mix together tomatoes, red onion, bell pepper, salsa, salt and pepper. Serve the fish with the salsa mixture in warm corn tortillas.

Time: 20 minutes.

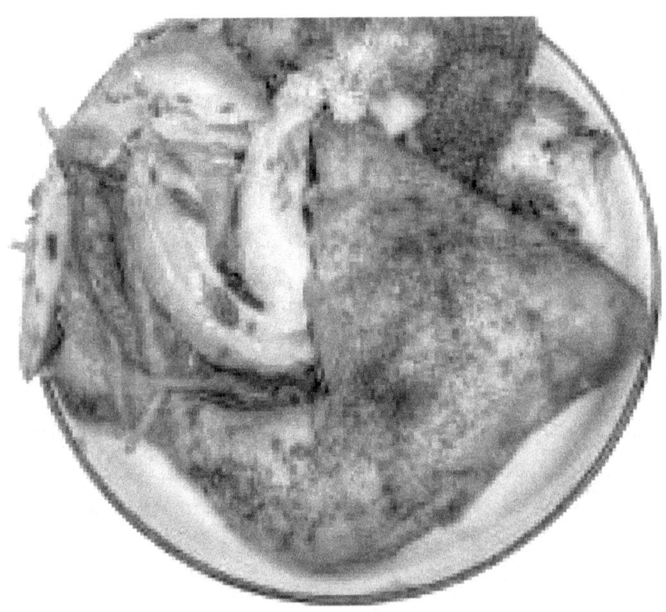

CHAPTER FIVE

Soup Recipes

Carrot and Coriander Soup:

Ingredients:

2 tablespoons olive oil, 1 onion, 2 cloves of garlic, 2 large carrots, 1 litre vegetable stock, 2 tablespoons coriander leaves, salt and pepper

Method of Preparation:

In a big saucepan, heat the oil. After adding, sauté the onion and garlic for a few minutes, or until softened. The carrots are then added, and cooking time is increased. Bring to a boil after adding the stock.

The carrots should be soft after 20 minutes of simmering at a reduced heat. Turn off the heat and use a hand blender to combine. Add the coriander and season to your liking.

Time of Preparation: 30 minutes

Broccoli and Cheese Soup:

Ingredients:

2 tablespoons butter, 1 onion, 2 cloves of garlic, 2 tablespoons plain flour, 1 litre vegetable stock, 2 heads of broccoli, 2 tablespoons cream, 1/2 cup grated cheddar cheese, salt and pepper

Method of Preparation:

Melt the butter in a large saucepan. Once added, cook the onion and garlic until soft. Add the flour and stir-fry for one to two minutes. Pour the stock in gradually while stirring, then bring to a boil. For 15 minutes, simmer on a lower heat.

After adding the broccoli, simmer for an additional 10 minutes. Turn off the heat and use a hand blender to combine. Stir through the cream and cheese and season to taste.

Time of Preparation: 30 minutes

Mushroom and Barley Soup:

Ingredients:

2 tablespoons olive oil, 1 onion, 2 cloves of garlic, 250g mushrooms, 2 tablespoons pearl barley, 1 litre vegetable stock, salt and pepper

Method of Preparation:

In a big saucepan, heat the oil. For a few minutes, add the onion and garlic and heat until softened. Add the mushrooms and continue to cook for a few more minutes. Bring to a boil after adding the stock. Reduce the heat and simmer for 20 minutes or until the mushrooms are tender. Add the pearl barley and simmer for 10 minutes more. Turn off the heat and add salt to your liking.

Time of Preparation: 30 minutes

Lentil and Tomato Soup:

Ingredients:

2 tablespoons olive oil, 1 onion, 2 cloves of garlic, 1 carrot, 1 celery stick, 200g red lentils, 1 litre vegetable stock, 1 tin chopped tomatoes, salt and pepper

Method of Preparation:

In a big saucepan, heat the oil. After adding, sauté the onion and garlic for a few minutes, or until softened. After adding, simmer the carrot and celery for an additional few minute. Bring to a boil the stock, lentils, and other ingredients.

The lentils should be soft after 20 minutes of simmering at a low heat. Simmer for a further 10 minutes after adding the chopped tomatoes. Turn off the heat and add salt to your liking.

Time of Preparation: 30 minutes

Sweet Potato and Coconut Soup:
Ingredients:

2 tablespoons coconut oil, 1 onion, 2 cloves of garlic, 2 large sweet potatoes, 1 litre vegetable stock, 1 tin coconut milk, salt and pepper

Method of Preparation:

Heat the coconut oil in a large saucepan. After adding, sauté the onion and garlic for a few minutes, or until softened. Add the sweet potatoes and cook for a few minutes more. Bring to a boil after adding the stock. Reduce the heat and simmer for 20 minutes or until the sweet potatoes are tender. Turn off the heat and use a hand blender to combine. Stir through the coconut milk and season.

Time of Preparation: 30 minutes

French Onion Soup:

Ingredients:

2 tablespoons olive oil, 4 large onions, 2 cloves of garlic, 1 litre vegetable stock, 4 slices of wholegrain bread, 2 tablespoons grated cheese, salt and pepper

Method of Preparation:

In a big saucepan, heat the oil. Add the onions and garlic and cook for 15 minutes or until softened and golden. Add the stock and then bring to a boil. Simmer for ten minutes on low heat. Place the bread on top of the soup and sprinkle over the cheese. Grill until melted and golden. Turn off the heat and add salt to your liking.

Time of Preparation: 30 minutes

Spinach and Potato Soup:

Ingredients:

2 tablespoons olive oil, 1 onion, 2 cloves of garlic, 2 large potatoes, 1 litre vegetable stock, 200g spinach, salt and pepper

Method of Preparation:

In a big saucepan, heat the oil. After adding, sauté the onion and garlic for a few minutes, or until softened. Next add the potatoes and simmer for a further few minutes. Bring to a boil after adding the stock. The potatoes should be cooked after 20 minutes of simmering at a reduced heat. Add the spinach, cook it for a further five minutes. Turn off the heat and use a hand blender to combine. Season to taste.

Time of Preparation: 30 minutes

Avocado and Cucumber Soup:

Ingredients:

2 tablespoons olive oil, 1 onion, 2 cloves of garlic, 2 ripe avocados, 2 large cucumbers, 1 litre vegetable stock, 2 tablespoons yoghurt, salt and pepper

Method of Preparation:

In a big saucepan, heat the oil. After adding, sauté the onion and garlic for a few minutes, or until softened. Cucumbers and avocados are then added, and cooking time is increased. Add the stock and then bring to a boil. Simmer for ten minutes on low heat. Turn off the heat and use a hand blender to combine. Yogurt should be incorporated after flavoring to taste.

Time of Preparation: 20 minutes

Cauliflower and Cheese Soup:

Ingredients:

2 tablespoons butter, 1 onion, 2 cloves of garlic, 1 large cauliflower, 1 litre vegetable stock, 2 tablespoons cream, 1/2 cup grated cheddar cheese, salt and pepper

Method of Preparation:

Melt the butter in a large saucepan. After being added, cook the onion and garlic until they are soft. Cook for a further couple minutes after adding the cauliflower. Add the stock and then bring to a boil. After turning down the heat, simmer the cauliflower for 15 minutes, or until it is soft. Turn off the heat and use a hand blender to combine. Stir through the cream and cheese and season to taste.

Time of Preparation: 25 minutes

Tomato and Basil Soup:

Ingredients:

2 tablespoons olive oil, 1 onion, 2 cloves of garlic, 1 litre vegetable stock, 2 tins chopped tomatoes, 4 tablespoons chopped fresh basil, salt and pepper

Method of Preparation:

Heat the oil in a large saucepan for a few minutes, add the onion and garlic and heat until softened. Bring to a boil after adding the stock and tomatoes. For 15 minutes, simmer on a lower heat. Turn off the heat and use a hand blender to combine. Add the basil and season to taste after stirring. ***Time of Preparation: 20 minutes***

CHAPTER SIX

Salad Recipes

Avocado, Grilled Chicken, and Spinach Salad:

Ingredients:

- 2 boneless and skinless chicken breasts

- 2 tablespoons olive oil, divided

- 1/2 teaspoon garlic powder

- 2 tablespoons balsamic vinegar

- 2 tablespoons honey

- 1/4 teaspoon freshly ground black pepper

- 4 cups baby spinach

- 1 avocado, diced

- 2 tablespoons chopped walnuts

- 2 tablespoons crumbled feta cheese

Method of Preparation:

1. Preheat the grill to medium-high heat.

2. Brush each chicken breast with 1 tablespoon olive oil and sprinkle with garlic powder.

3. The chicken breasts should be cooked through after grilling for 4–5 minutes on each side.

4. Meanwhile, in a small bowl, whisk together the remaining 1 tablespoon olive oil, balsamic vinegar, honey, and black pepper.

5. In a large bowl, combine the spinach, avocado, walnuts, and feta cheese.

6. Add the grilled chicken and the dressing, and toss to combine.

Time of Preparation: 20 minutes.

Beetroot, Feta, and Apple Salad:

Ingredients:

- 2 large beetroots, cooked, peeled and diced

- 2 apples, diced

- 2 tablespoons olive oil

- 2 tablespoons lemon juice

- 2 tablespoons honey

- 1/4 teaspoon freshly ground black pepper

- 4 cups baby spinach

- 1/2 cup feta cheese, crumbled

- 2 tablespoons chopped walnuts

Method of Preparation:

1. In a large bowl, combine the beetroot, apples, olive oil, lemon juice, honey, and black pepper.

2. Add the spinach, feta cheese, and walnuts and toss to combine.

Time of Preparation: 15 minutes.

Kale, Quinoa, and Sweet Potato Salad:
Ingredients:

- 2 sweet potatoes, diced

- 2 tablespoons olive oil

- 1/2 teaspoon garlic powder

- 1/4 teaspoon freshly ground black pepper

- 4 cups kale, chopped

- 1/2 cup cooked quinoa

- 2 tablespoons chopped walnuts

- 2 tablespoons crumbled feta cheese

Method of Preparation:

1. Preheat the oven to 400°F.

2. Spread the diced sweet potatoes on a baking sheet and drizzle with the olive oil. Sprinkle with the garlic powder and black pepper.

3. Bake for 20 minutes, or until tender.

4. Meanwhile, in a large bowl, combine the kale, quinoa, walnuts, and feta cheese.

5. Add the roasted sweet potatoes and toss to combine.

Time of Preparation: 25 minutes.

Carrot, Raisin, and Chickpea Salad:

Ingredients:

- 2 cups cooked chickpeas

- 1/4 cup olive oil

- 2 tablespoons apple cider vinegar

- 2 tablespoons honey

- 1/4 teaspoon freshly ground black pepper

- 4 cups baby spinach

- 2 carrots, grated

- 1/4 cup raisins

- 2 tablespoons chopped walnuts

Method of Preparation:

1. In a small bowl, whisk together the olive oil, apple cider vinegar, honey, and black pepper.

2. In a large bowl, combine the chickpeas, spinach, carrots, raisins, and walnuts.

3. Add the dressing and toss to combine.

Time of Preparation: 10 minutes.

Cucumber, Tomato, and Feta Salad:

Ingredients:

- 2 cucumbers, diced

- 2 tomatoes, diced

- 2 tablespoons olive oil

- 2 tablespoons lemon juice

- 2 tablespoons honey

- 1/4 teaspoon freshly ground black pepper

- 4 cups baby spinach

- 1/2 cup feta cheese, crumbled

- 2 tablespoons chopped walnuts

Method of Preparation:

1. In a small bowl, whisk together the olive oil, lemon juice, honey, and black pepper.

2. In a large bowl, combine the cucumbers, tomatoes, spinach, feta cheese, and walnuts.

3. Add the dressing and toss to combine.

Time of Preparation: 10 minutes.

Broccoli, Avocado, and Quinoa Salad:

Ingredients:

- 2 cups cooked quinoa

- 2 tablespoons olive oil

- 2 tablespoons lemon juice

- 2 tablespoons honey

- 1/4 teaspoon freshly ground black pepper

- 2 cups broccoli florets

- 1 avocado, diced

- 2 tablespoons chopped walnuts

Method of Preparation:

1. In a small bowl, whisk together the olive oil, lemon juice, honey, and black pepper.

2. In a large bowl, combine the quinoa, broccoli, avocado, and walnuts.

3. Add the dressing and toss to combine.

Time of Preparation: 10 minutes.

Arugula, Orange, and Almond Salad:

Ingredients:

- 2 oranges, peeled and diced

- 2 tablespoons olive oil

- 2 tablespoons orange juice

- 2 tablespoons honey

- 1/4 teaspoon freshly ground black pepper

- 4 cups baby arugula

- 2 tablespoons chopped almonds

Method of Preparation:

1. In a small bowl, whisk together the olive oil, orange juice, honey, and black pepper.

2. In a large bowl, combine the oranges, arugula, and almonds.

3. Add the dressing and toss to combine.

Time of Preparation: 10 minutes.

Egg, Bacon, and Avocado Salad:

Ingredients:

- 4 large eggs

- 4 strips bacon

- 2 tablespoons olive oil

- 2 tablespoons lemon juice

- 2 tablespoons honey

- 1/4 teaspoon freshly ground black pepper

- 4 cups baby spinach

- 1 avocado, diced

Method of Preparation:

1. Preheat the oven to 400°F.

2. Place the eggs and bacon on a baking sheet and bake for 12-15 minutes, or until the bacon is cooked and the eggs are set.

3. Meanwhile, in a small bowl, whisk together the olive oil, lemon juice, honey, and black pepper.

4. In a large bowl, combine the spinach and avocado.

5. Add the cooked eggs and bacon and the dressing, and toss to combine.

Time of Preparation: 20 minutes.

Spinach, Cheddar, and Pear Salad:
Ingredients:

- 2 pears, diced

- 2 tablespoons olive oil

- 2 tablespoons balsamic vinegar

- 2 tablespoons honey

- 1/4 teaspoon freshly ground black pepper

- 4 cups baby spinach

- 1/2 cup cheddar cheese, shredded

- 2 tablespoons chopped walnuts

Method of Preparation:

1. In a small bowl, whisk together the olive oil, balsamic vinegar, honey, and black pepper.

2. In a large bowl, combine the pears, spinach, cheddar cheese, and walnuts.

3. Add the dressing and toss to combine.

Time of Preparation: 10 minutes.

Cabbage, Cucumber, and Feta Salad:

Ingredients:

- 1/2 head cabbage, shredded

- 2 cucumbers, diced

- 2 tablespoons olive oil

- 2 tablespoons lemon juice

- 2 tablespoons honey

- 1/4 teaspoon freshly ground black pepper

- 4 cups baby spinach

- 1/2 cup feta cheese, crumbled

Method of Preparation:

1. In a small bowl, whisk together the olive oil, lemon juice, honey, and black pepper.

2. In a large bowl, combine the cabbage, cucumbers, spinach, and feta cheese.

3. Add the dressing and toss to combine.

Time of Preparation: 10 minutes.

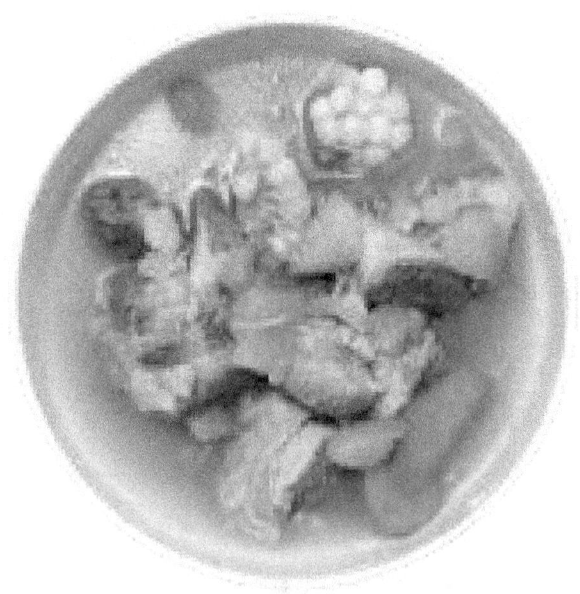

CHAPTER SEVEN

Sea-Food Recipes

Baked Salmon with Ginger and Garlic

Ingredients:

4 salmon fillets, 2 cloves of garlic, 2 tablespoons of grated ginger, 2 tablespoons of olive oil, Salt and pepper to taste

Method of Preparation:

Preheat oven to 375 degrees Fahrenheit. Put the salmon fillets in a baking dish that has been buttered. Mix the garlic, ginger, olive oil, salt, and pepper in a small bowl. Overlay the salmon fillets with the mixture.

Bake the salmon for 15 to 20 minutes, or until it is thoroughly done.

Time of Preparation: 20 minutes

Grilled Tuna Steaks with Cucumber Salsa

Ingredients:

4 tuna steaks, 1 cucumber, 1 red onion, 1 red bell pepper, 2 tablespoons of olive oil, 2 tablespoons of red wine vinegar, Salt and pepper to taste

Method of Preparation:

Preheat a grill or grill pan to medium-high. Place the tuna steaks on the grill and cook for 3 minutes per side, or until cooked through. Meanwhile, dice the cucumber, red onion, and bell pepper. Combine the olive oil, red wine vinegar, salt, and pepper in a small bowl. Toss the vegetables with the dressing. Serve the tuna steaks with the cucumber salsa.

Time of Preparation: 15 minutes

Shrimp and Vegetable Stir Fry

Ingredients:

1 tablespoon of olive oil, 1 pound of shrimp, 1 cup of broccoli florets, 1 red bell pepper, 1 cup of sliced mushrooms, 2 cloves of garlic, 2 tablespoons of soy sauce

Method of Preparation:

In a large skillet over medium-high heat, warm the olive oil. Cook for 2 minutes after adding the shrimp. Add the broccoli, bell pepper, mushrooms, and garlic and cook for another 5 minutes, or until the vegetables are tender. Add the soy sauce, stir, and simmer for one more minute. Serve over cooked rice.

Time of Preparation: 10 minutes

Fish Tacos with Avocado Cream Sauce

Ingredients:

1 pound of cod fillets, 1 teaspoon of smoked paprika, 1 teaspoon of garlic powder, 1 teaspoon of chili powder, 1 teaspoon of cumin, 8 taco shells, 1 avocado, ½ cup of sour cream, 1 lime, Salt and pepper to taste

Method of Preparation:

Preheat oven to 375 degrees Fahrenheit. Line a baking sheet with parchment paper. Combine the cumin, garlic powder, chili powder, and smoked paprika in a small bowl. Rub the mixture evenly over the cod fillets. Bake the fish for 15 to 20 minutes, or until it is thoroughly done.

Meanwhile, mash the avocado in a small bowl. Stir in the sour cream, juice of the lime, salt, and pepper. To assemble the tacos, place the cod in the taco shells and top with the avocado cream sauce.

Time of Preparation: 25 minutes

Baked Cod with Roasted Tomatoes

Ingredients:

4 cod fillets, 1 pint of cherry tomatoes, 2 tablespoons of olive oil, 2 cloves of garlic, 2 tablespoons of fresh parsley, Salt and pepper to taste

Method of Preparation:

Preheat oven to 375 degrees Fahrenheit. Cod fillets should be placed in a greased baking dish. Arrange the cherry tomatoes around the cod. Drizzle the olive oil over the top. Sprinkle the garlic and parsley over the entire dish. Season with salt and pepper. Bake the fish for 15 to 20 minutes, or until it is thoroughly done.

Time of Preparation: 20 minutes

Crab Cakes with Lemon Aioli

Ingredients:

1 pound of lump crab meat, 2 cloves of garlic, ¼ cup of diced red onion, ½ cup of panko breadcrumbs, 2 eggs, 2 tablespoons of mayonnaise, 2 tablespoons of Dijon mustard, 2 tablespoons of lemon juice, 2 tablespoons of olive oil, Salt and pepper to taste

Method of Preparation:

In a large bowl, mix together the crab meat, garlic, red onion, breadcrumbs, eggs, mayonnaise, mustard, lemon juice, salt, and pepper. Put the mixture on a prepared baking sheet and shape it into patties. Drizzle the olive oil over the top of the patties. Bake for 15 to 20 minutes, or until golden brown, at 375 degrees Fahrenheit.

Meanwhile, mix together the remaining mayonnaise, lemon juice, and salt and pepper. Crab cakes should be served with lemon aioli.

Time of Preparation: 25 minutes

Grilled Halibut with Parsley Salsa

Ingredients:

4 halibut fillets, 2 tablespoons of olive oil, 1 cup of fresh parsley, ½ cup of diced tomatoes, 1 clove of garlic, 2 tablespoons of red wine vinegar, Salt and pepper to taste

Method of Preparation:

Preheat a grill or grill pan to medium-high. Season the halibut fillets after brushing them with olive oil. Place the fillets on the grill and cook for 3-4 minutes per side, or until cooked through. Meanwhile, mix together the parsley, tomatoes, garlic, red wine vinegar, salt, and pepper in a small bowl. Serve the halibut fillets with the parsley salsa.

Time of Preparation: 15 minutes

Shrimp Scampi with Garlic Toast

Ingredients:

1 pound of shrimp, 2 tablespoons of butter, 2 cloves of garlic, 2 tablespoons of white wine, 2 tablespoons of lemon juice, 4 slices of French bread, 2 tablespoons of olive oil

Method of Preparation:

Heat the butter in a large skillet over medium-high heat. Add the shrimp and cook for three minutes. Add the garlic, white wine, and lemon juice and cook for another 2 minutes. Meanwhile, brush the French bread slices with olive oil. Toast on a baking sheet in the oven at 375 degrees Fahrenheit for 10 minutes, or until golden brown. Serve the shrimp scampi with the garlic toast.

Time of Preparation: 15 minutes

Clam Chowder

Ingredients:

4 cups of clam juice, 2 cups of potatoes, ¼ cup of diced onion, 1 cup of diced celery, 2 tablespoons of butter, 2 tablespoons of all-purpose flour, 1 cup of half-and-half, 1 6-ounce can of chopped clams, Salt and pepper to taste

Method of Preparation:

In a large pot, bring the clam juice to a boil. Add the potatoes, onion, and celery and simmer until the vegetables are tender, about 15 minutes. Melt the butter over medium heat in a separate pan. After adding the flour, simmer for two minutes. Add the half-and-half gradually while stirring, then simmer.

Add the half-and-half mixture to the vegetable-filled stew and stir. Salt and pepper the clams before adding them. Simmer for 10 minutes, or until the chowder is thickened.

Time of Preparation: 30 minutes

Baked Lobster Tails

Ingredients:

4 lobster tails, 4 tablespoons of butter, 2 cloves of garlic, 2 tablespoons of lemon juice, Salt and pepper to taste

Method of Preparation:

Preheat oven to 375 degrees Fahrenheit. Place the lobster tails in a greased baking dish. In a small bowl, mix together the butter, garlic, lemon juice, salt, and pepper. Spread the mixture over the top of the lobster tails. Bake for 15-20 minutes, or until the lobster is cooked through.

Time of Preparation: 20 minutes

30 Days Meal Plan

	Breakfast	Lunch	Dinner
Day 1	Oatmeal with fresh berries, a glass of orange juice	Lentil soup and a side salad	Baked salmon with roasted vegetables
Day 2	Scrambled eggs and whole-wheat toast	Tuna and white bean salad	Grilled chicken with steamed broccoli
Day 3	Yogurt and fruit parfait	Turkey and vegetable wrap	Baked cod with roasted sweet potatoes
Day 4	Omelet with vegetables	Quinoa and black bean salad	Roasted turkey with mashed potatoes
Day 5	Whole-wheat toast with peanut butter	Grilled cheese sandwich	Baked tilapia with steamed spinach
Day 6	Smoothie with banana, berries, and almond milk	Bean and cheese burrito	Grilled pork chop with roasted vegetables
Day 7	Oatmeal with blueberries and walnuts	Soup and salad	Baked chicken with roasted potatoes
Day 8	Scrambled eggs and whole-wheat toast	Chicken salad sandwich	Grilled salmon with asparagus
Day 9	Greek yogurt with granola and berries	Hummus and vegetable wrap	Baked tilapia with roasted vegetables

Day 10	Whole-grain waffles with yogurt and fruit	Lentil soup and a side salad	Grilled steak with mashed potatoes
Day 11	Omelet with vegetables	Turkey and avocado sandwich	Baked cod with steamed broccoli
Day 12	Smoothie with banana, spinach, and almond milk	Quinoa and black bean salad	Grilled chicken with roasted sweet potatoes
Day 13	Whole-wheat toast with peanut butter	Bean and cheese burrito	Baked salmon with steamed spinach
Day 14	Oatmeal with fresh berries and a glass of orange juice	Tuna and white bean salad	Roasted turkey with roasted vegetables
Day 15	Yogurt and fruit parfait	Grilled cheese sandwich	Baked tilapia with mashed potatoes
Day 16	Scrambled eggs and whole-wheat toast	Hummus and vegetable wrap	Grilled pork chop with asparagus
Day 17	Smoothie with banana, berries, and almond milk	Lentil Soup and salad	Baked chicken with roasted potatoes
Day 18	Omelet with vegetables	Chicken salad sandwich	Grilled salmon with roasted vegetables
Day 19	Greek yogurt with granola and berries	Quinoa and black bean salad	Baked tilapia with steamed broccoli

Day 20	Whole-grain waffles with yogurt and fruit	Lentil soup and a side salad	Grilled steak with mashed potatoes
Day 21	Oatmeal with blueberries and walnuts	Turkey and avocado sandwich	Baked cod with roasted sweet potatoes
Day 22	Whole-wheat toast with peanut butter	Bean and cheese burrito	Grilled chicken with steamed spinach
Day 23	Smoothie with banana, spinach, and almond milk	Tuna and white bean salad	Roasted turkey with roasted vegetables
Day 24	Yogurt and fruit parfait	Hummus and vegetable wrap	Baked salmon with mashed potatoes
Day 25	Omelet with vegetables	Soup and salad	Grilled pork chop with asparagus
Day 26	Scrambled eggs and whole-wheat toast	Chicken salad sandwich	Baked tilapia with roasted vegetables
Day 27	Greek yogurt with granola and berries	Quinoa and black bean salad	Grilled steak with steamed broccoli
Day 28	Whole wheat toast with natural peanut butter	Turkey and avocado sandwich	Baked cod with mashed potatoes
Day 29	Whole-grain waffles with yogurt and fruit	Turkey burger and a side of sweet potato fries	Grilled chicken with roasted sweet potatoes

Day 30	Smoothie with banana, berries, and almond milk	Spinach salad with grilled chicken, tomatoes and cucumbers	Baked salmon with roasted vegetables

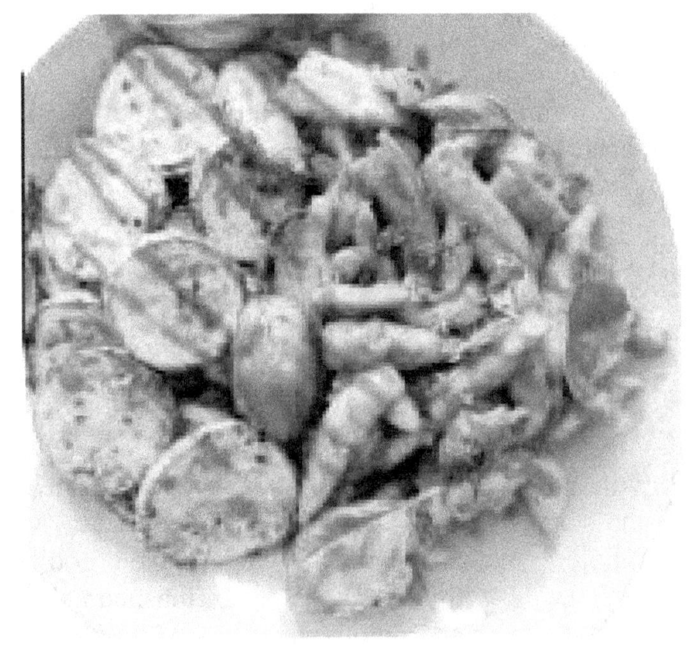

CONCLUSION

In conclusion, it is clear that the practice of providing one meal a day for seniors is an effective way to ensure their nutritional needs are met. The meal provides the elderly with the necessary vitamins and minerals, as well as a sense of community and socialization.

It also helps to reduce the risk of malnutrition, which is a very real concern for the elderly population. Additionally, providing just one meal a day helps to keep the costs down for both the senior and the care providers.

The benefits of providing one meal a day for seniors are numerous, and the potential for a healthier, more enjoyable life for the elderly is great. By providing a balanced meal every day, seniors can maintain their independence and remain active and involved in their communities. It is a cost-effective way to ensure their nutritional needs are met and to help them remain healthy and vibrant.

The practice of providing one meal a day for seniors can make a positive impact on the lives of the elderly. It is a simple, yet effective way to ensure their nutritional needs are met and to help them remain healthy and vibrant. This practice is a valuable one and should be embraced by all who care for the elderly.

Just like my grandpa, every senior deserves a good life with the required nutrition. Therefore, I would like to urge everyone to play their part in providing one meal a day for seniors in their own way. With our collective effort, we can make sure that no senior will have to worry about their nutrition and health.

SPEAK TO YOUR BODY

I am made whole

I'm living my best life

I will take control of my health and make healthy choices

My blood pressure is normal and I am feeling vibrant and strong

I am confident in my ability to make positive changes in my life that will benefit my overall well-being

I honor my body and recognize the power of self-care

I respect and love myself and I know that I am capable of living a life of good health and wellness.

I believe in Jesus and in the power of His resurrection to bring healing and strength to my body.

I believe He died and rose again to provide me with the power to overcome any health challenges that come my way.

I accept Him as my Lord and saviour and I trust that He will guide me on my journey to wellness. Amen